WHAT IS ARNICA?

Why Arnica Montana is the #1 Best-Selling Homeopathic Remedy in the World

RUTH ELSTON

BETTER LIFE BOOKS

To a healthy, natural life.

CONTENTS

ACKNOWLEDGMENTS

A big thank you to Tom at Better Life Books.

Also, to Lynne and Juanita for their help and suggestions.

Introduction

I have used Arnica for at least twenty years and have been an enthusiastic promoter of its healing and pain relieving benefits for almost as long.

Arnica is one of the safest of all homeopathic remedies that can be used without the guidance of a doctor. Arnica is gentle, safe and has none of the nasty side effects that so many drugs do. How could I not be an enthusiast!

Please give this amazing homeopathic remedy an honest try and self treat those everyday ailments that hardly justify the expense of a visit to the doctor.

I have kept a supply of Arnica with me for as long as I can remember and as you will see in some of the stories that follow, I usually carry a spare bottle or two to give to friends.

Many of the little booklets I used to give to my friends over the years now seem to be out of print. Hence, my small book – *"What is Arnica?"*

About Arnica Montana

Arnica, also known as Arnica Montana, is the most loved and the most widely used remedy in all of homeopathy. It could even be said that it is the success of Arnica that has led to the success of homeopathy.

The plant (a beautiful yellow/orange, daisy-like flower) has been used for medicinal purposes for thousands of years. More than one hundred prescription drugs are made from the herb in Germany alone, (where it is known as 'Fallkraut') and it is one of the most popular holistic remedies in all of Europe.

Arnica is the #1 best-selling homeopathic remedy in the world today. Why? Because it works! Arnica is magical, miraculous and wonderful.

Arnica has been healing people for centuries, far longer than pharmaceutical companies have been manufacturing painkillers.

One of the many wonderful things about homeopathic Arnica is that it can never cause harm and yet brings relief to so many health problems. There are precautions you should take with herbal preparations of Arnica - it should never be ingested and never applied to open wounds - but it is impossible to overdose on homeopathic remedies because the dilution is so great.

The only 'harm' in taking too much of homeopathic Arnica would be to reduce its effectiveness. That 'less is more' is one of the most difficult aspects of homeopathy to grasp.

Discover for yourself the potency and power of the minimum dose!

Arnica for Sleep & Overtiredness

I love my sleep, and I'm guessing that after all the stresses of even a normal day, you like your sleep too. But what do you do when you can't sleep?

Thousands of people all over the world are suffering from insomnia or overtiredness. They experience non-restorative sleep, early morning awakenings, difficulty in maintaining sleep or difficulty in initiating sleep.

There are three types of insomnia: transient or short term insomnia, chronic or constant insomnia and intermittent insomnia. Arnica is best for transient insomnia caused by overexertion or stressful events.

It's wonderful for jet lag for example. Last year I flew to New Zealand with my husband and his business colleagues. The journey took well over 24 hours with stops in several different times zones. Both my husband and I took Arnica tablets before we left, and twice on the flight, and neither of us felt any jet lag. Remarkable when compared to others in the party, many of whom took several days to recover.

I never travel anywhere without my Arnica and my homeopathic first aid kit.

After a stressful day take a bath with an Arnica bath soak, and you will sleep like a log. To recover from tiredness brought on by overstrained muscles, try one pill of Arnica 30 at bedtime.

The main causes of insomnia are advanced age, depression, a secondary medical problem, sleep apnea, overuse of caffeine, anxiety and stress.

Most individuals suffering from insomnia and overtiredness are given sleeping pills, but these aren't always the best option. Sleeping pills treat the symptom, not the cause, and they come with numerous side effects. They can affect your memory, judgment and consciousness and, above all, they can create dependency. Arnica is totally non habit-forming.

There are many homeopathic remedies for treating sleeping problems, of which Arnica is only one. A homeopath or health store will be able to recommend other natural solutions.

My mother told me that when she was young she had chronic sleeping problems. She was constantly overtired from raising quite a large family and still having to work late in the evenings at a part time nursing job. Despite her tiredness she found it difficult to fall asleep and during the night she awoke often. In the morning she was even more tired than before she went to sleep! She tried different medicines from her doctor but they just made her feel worse. In fact, she even tried some natural remedies suggested to her by friends and colleagues, but none of them worked for her. Fortunately, one day a friend told her she had read about the wonderful benefits of Arnica and bought her some to try as one last remedy. She started taking the Arnica pills she had been given and after a few days she started feeling better. She began to fall asleep much more quickly, slept all night and felt completely rested in the morning. Once the overtiredness was gone she immediately regained her energy. I must say, the Arnica given by her friend not only proved a blessing to my mother but to the whole family!

Arnica is also suitable for sleep problems caused by nightmares as well as for sleeplessness triggered by weariness and over - exertion of the mind.

In addition, Arnica is beneficial for individuals struggling to sleep due to aches or muscle pain. You know the feeling: no matter what position you lie in you just can't get comfortable and the bed feels too hard. I find just one little Arnica pill reduces the discomfort very quickly.

My son used to be a sales rep and his job meant he often had to travel from one town to another, sleeping in different beds as he went. During a 'phone call home he told me he couldn't wait to get back to his own bed to get a decent night's sleep again and I reminded him to try a dose of Arnica at bedtime. Sure enough, it worked and although he still prefers his own bed he no longer has trouble sleeping in others!

So anyone who has to travel for a living (long distance truck drivers for example), or travels for fun (backpackers and campers spring to mind), will find Arnica helps them to get a good night's sleep in even the most uncomfortable circumstances. Not only will it make a hard bed seem softer, it will reduce the anxiety and tension that so often accompanies our exposure to the unfamiliar.

Arnica restores the sleep balance and helps you relax. For anyone with sleep problems I would recommend taking Arnica 30 twice daily, with the last dose taken just before bedtime.

Sleep and Recover!

Arnica for Pets & Animals

The successful use of Arnica on people can equally be applied to pets and animals. More and more vets have discovered this and are now using Arnica in their surgeries and prescribing to their clients.

This is a wonderful development but we have to understand that it is more difficult to detect when and where to apply Arnica to an animal. After all they can't tell you how they feel and where exactly they hurt.

One of the indications that Arnica is required is when the injured animal is afraid of being touched. It might not be surprising after an accident, of course, but still not every injured animal reacts in the same way. Some can be frightened or aggressive and some just very subdued. The fear of being further hurt can make the animal shrink away from touch or being approached. It's in exactly these instances that Arnica is the best remedy.

When it is clear the injury is to muscles or soft tissues, first give Arnica pills to restore calm and then Arnica ointment can be applied. Arnica pills should be given in all cases of shock.

Many veterinarians now give animals Arnica tablets in order to diminish the emotional stress before and after a surgical intervention. An Arnica cream is often used on the area where the animal has suffered the trauma.

Some of the most common complaints in pets are just the same as humans i.e. sprains, sore muscles, possible arthritis, and bruises.

It's important to remember that if you want to use an Arnica gel to help your pets, then just as in the case with humans you should never put it on an open wound. For broken skin and lesions, homeopathic pills are better advised.

There are two easy ways to give Arnica to a dog or cat. You can put a single pill into the mouth of the pet and make sure they swallow it. The pills are very tiny and most pets swallow them willingly.

For pets that won't take a pill, simply put the pill it into a small amount of water and stir, then give just a teaspoon of the liquid to the pet. Don't worry if the pellet hasn't dissolved.

As with human injuries, just one or two doses should be enough and that dosage applies to pets of all sizes.

My very good friend Pat has been a bit of a skeptic when it comes to using homeopathy, but when she couldn't find out what was troubling her beloved dog she was prepared to give my suggestion a try. This is what she told me about her little Jack Russell terrier:

"Spot was so sick, he would shiver as if trembling in pain and he would hardly eat anything. The poor thing could barely walk and when he did, his tail was tucked between his legs. I was so concerned I took him to the vet, who said he couldn't find anything physically wrong. He suggested that Spot was pining for John (her son who had recently left for college). John had been gone for a few weeks and the symptoms had only recently started - so I didn't think it was that - I still thought it was allergies or an infection. But I followed your advice and gave him some Arnica. Within a day he was bouncing around again like a puppy! He's got all his appetite back, there's no more trembling and I'm sure it's saved me a small fortune in further vet bills".

I had discussed the use of Arnica on pets with Sally, a friend of my daughter, when we met some months ago. This is what she told me in a recent email;

"My 2 year old Labrador (Spike) had a collision with a motorbike a couple of weeks ago and suffered really bad bruising. Although the vet assured me that nothing was broken his back leg was obviously very sore. There was quite a lump and if you looked carefully you could see the skin was turning purple. The bruising reminded me of what you had told me about Arnica. It turns out our vet stocks a whole range of natural products, and he also recommended Arnica. He gave us a gel that contained Arnica and I rubbed this onto the skin every 8 hours as directed. In only a couple of days the lump and bruise had completely gone and Spike was running and playing again. It was certainly worth trying this new (to me) treatment, and I'm so glad you told me

about it. Have just bought a small range of Arnica products for the family, just in case. It's not just Spike who has accidents round my place – the kids are worse than the dogs!"

Sally was right about the kids. Children and pets suffer many painful tumbles and bump into things we adults can avoid. I recommend a dose of Arnica to sooth the tears and another dose if there is bruising. I know of several teachers who keep Arnica handy for all the falls and scrapes on the school playground.

Arnica is extremely helpful for pets that have to travel. My daughter takes her dogs with her on holiday and often has them in the car for very long distances. She finds giving them Arnica before the journey keeps them calm and relaxed throughout.

It is even more helpful for pets that have to travel alone. One can only imagine the fear and anxiety caused to animals travelling unaccompanied in aircraft holds, or in baggage compartments on trains. I find Arnica works much better than tranquilizers in these circumstances.

Save money on veterinary bills and keep your beloved pet happy, pain free and healthy. Use Arnica!

Arnica in Sport

Everyone actively involved in sports or exercise needs to learn how Arnica helps speed up the recovery of everything from tired muscles to bone crushing injuries. Injuries in sport are common and it's not only in contact sports that they result in some form of muscle strain, shock, bruising, and damaged bones.

Not surprising then that Arnica is becoming the 'first out of the medicine bag' for sports trainers and coaches all over the world. Gone are the days of a sponge soaked in ice cold water (though believe me that treatment still works)!

Colin Jackson, the 110m hurdles world champion from 1992 to 1994, in an interview is quoted as saying about his sport injuries: *"I'd use anything that would get me back on the track as quickly as possible. Acupuncture was great, and some homeopathy worked remarkably well: Arnica tablets were really effective."*

As we know all too well from recent controversies, many sportsmen and women will use anything to get back to fitness. The real added value of Arnica in sports is its non-doping healing quality that makes it inconsequential to doping restrictions.

For muscle soreness, take one tablet of Arnica three times daily. Ideally you should take 24 hours before exercise and continue taking it after the exercise until the muscles recover and feel less sore. Arnica gel, lotions or creams can be applied on sore areas two to three times a day until soreness subsides.

All athletes can use Arnica to recover from sore and stiff muscles after strenuous workouts or competitions. For example horse riders can use it to help recover from their inevitable falls and bruises. Long distance runners, swimmers, cyclists, and triathletes should all use Arnica before races to improve their performance, minimize pain and reduce muscle cramp.

A twisted knee or ankle is a great risk for soccer players and physiotherapists at several English Premier League clubs now include Arnica to speed up the recovery of their players. Pierre Barrieu, a former head fitness coach for the United States Men's National Soccer Team is also said to be a strong advocate of using Arnica for the treatment of injured players.

Apart from a few doses of Arnica, sprains (to any part of the body) very rarely need any other form of treatment. Just to experience the speed of recovery from a sprained ankle for yourself will ensure you become a true believer in the healing power of Arnica.

Arnica can be used for reducing the pains and strains of all exercising – whether it's running a marathon, doing push-ups, working out in the gym or just enjoying digging around in the garden. Whether it's a blow to the eye from a baseball, a knock on the knee from a hockeystick, a kick on the shin or a punch on the jaw, treat them all with Arnica.

There are no side effects to homeopathic Arnica treatments and no interactions with other medicines. No wonder it's becoming so popular with sport professionals.

Many tennis players find Arnica Balm helpful during matches and then after a tough day on court, enjoy using Arnica bath soaks.

Many of the world's best cyclists use an Arnica Massage Oil during long competitive events. My son always uses Arnica Balm when his legs ache after cycling, to help him recover sooner.

Nowadays there are numerous remedies for sport injuries, but none of them are as beneficial and effective as Arnica. Sprains and other sport injuries can be healed with ointments containing Arnica. The ointment promotes natural recovery by dilating the blood vessels and allowing blood flow to return.

Whatever the injury and whatever the cause, the right dose of Arnica repeated at regular intervals will ease the pain and aid recovery every time.

In almost every case of sports injury, Arnica is truly the best remedy!

Teeth & Dental Troubles

When a dental surgeon extracts a tooth there is usually soreness and discomfort after the anesthetic wears off. Just a few doses of Arnica taken before and after dental work will remove any pain and soon have the mouth feeling comfortable again.

Modern dentistry is usually painless, but that doesn't alter the fact that many people still dread paying a visit to the dentist. Where Arnica is particularly helpful, is in reducing this fear and anxiety.

I believe that if dental surgeons kept a handy supply of Arnica in their surgeries they could help their patients relax and reduce any post surgery pain and discomfort.

Clarice, a good friend of mine, told me this story:

"When I was young I had tooth surgery and the doctor said that any pain wouldn't last long. Guess what, he was wrong! You know how they say that everything hurts when the weather changes? I'm 50 years old and believe me when it rains or it's just a bit chilly, my teeth hurt. I guess I'm too sensitive and that surgery finally got to my senses. The thing is, I wasn't in agony with the pain but I certainly didn't feel well. My teeth hurt, and I had a dull, nagging headache. I don't take

aspirin because of my allergy and other pain killers seemed to cause some unpleasant side effects. I was using Arnica Montana gel for knee pains but nobody had told me before you did, that I could also take Arnica tablets for toothache. Anyway, those Arnica 30's that you gave me when we were at your place really worked. My teeth are no longer sensitive, and my whole body feels so much better. Thank you, thank you, THANK YOU!"

Take Arnica before and after dental treatment!

Arnica for Injuries, Shock & Trauma

Arnica Montana is always the first choice remedy used by homeopaths to heal people affected by shock, trauma or injury to the body. No other remedy is so demonstrably effective.

Using Arnica to treat both the physical and emotional elements of shock and injury is one of the most researched and best documented of all its uses. To quote Phyllis Speight: *"It is in this area that Arnica shines most brilliantly"*.

Arnica Montana is the only remedy that heals both the trauma and shock, and the actual injury itself. All accidents, great or small, cause some degree of shock and Arnica can help in every case. That's why you should always carry an emergency bottle of Arnica with you.

A couple of years ago, I fell off the stepladders in our garage and landed on the hard cement floor. I was in shock, shaken, nauseous and barely able to move but managed to get to my jar of Arnica and take a pellet. After about 30 minutes I could move more freely and wasn't nauseous any longer. I sat down and started applying Arnica ointment on the problem areas. Amazingly the next day there was no bruising on my body.

Arnica salve, an old favorite of mine, is the best treatment for bruises and sprains. This miraculous ointment alleviates the pain, swelling and bruising triggered by muscle injuries. However, what is often more important than the bruising is the shock caused by the injury. Shock to the system can have long term consequences, often causing other ailments including depression. Alleviating the shock helps tremendously in the physical recovery from the injury.

Arnica is particularly effective for the accident victims who say, *"No, I'm fine, don't touch me, I'm OK, don't fuss,"* especially when it is obvious they do need help.

Basically, Arnica salve is a topical gel that can be rubbed onto the problem area. Besides the fact that it offers local pain relief, it also makes the body reabsorb the fluids and blood in the area. This greatly speeds up the healing process. The Arnica roots contain thymol, a substance that acts as a pain reliever and anti – inflammatory agent.

Various medical studies have shown that the expensive pharmaceutical treatments recommended by doctors are less effective in relieving muscular pain and healing bruising than Arnica.

Imagine bumping into something and getting one of those dark and sore bruises on your leg that usually lasts for days.... Wouldn't you like to rid yourself of the unsightly bruise as quickly as possible? Arnica is the single most powerful remedy against bruising!

Arnica is indeed a true wonder of nature!

Arnica & Common Ailments

Backache

I haven't tried it but some of my friends use a traditional Arnica formula, Hyland's BackAche, for the relief of lower back pain and swear by it.

Bites and Stings

When my daughter was 8 years old she experienced cellulitis as the result of a bug bite (might have been a spider). Her leg became quite swollen and there was some inflammation. Even in those days I preferred not to use antibiotics if I could avoid them, so I gave her one Arnica 30 pill. I then placed a few drops of Arnica tincture onto a cotton swab and applied it to her leg and also applied an ice pack. By morning, the inflammation was completely gone. She was able to freely move her leg and the redness had also subsided.

Eczema

My friend Clarice again:

"My daughter is now using Arnica for her eczema and is already seeing much improvement. I think I'm now a bigger fan of Arnica than you are!"

Frozen Shoulder

Pete's story:

"Truly amazing! I suffer from frozen shoulder, and after massaging in the Arnica rub, felt instant relief. Several massages later and I'm pretty sure the shoulder is healed."

Hemorrhoids

Dr Rudolf Fritz Weiss, MD (a famous German herbalist) recommends using 1-2 teaspoons of Arnica tincture per one pint of water as a wet compress to help relieve the symptoms associated with hemorrhoids.

Sore Feet

Another friend's story:

"I work in a department store and I'm on my feet for the best part of 9 hours a day, 6 days a week. I've been doing this job for over 20 years now, so my feet are a total mess. After you told me that Arnica was great for sore tired feet, I have started to use the gel as you recommended. Every day when I get home, I rub Arnica gel on my feet and then apply again before I go to bed. I'm more active at work, my feet are not in pain anymore, and now when I get home I don't feel that exhausted. I'm becoming a strong believer in all-natural remedies and I strongly recommend Arnica for all aches and pains."

Tennis Elbow

Jan's story:

"I have had bad tennis elbow and a sore muscle in my right arm for what seems like forever. I can't say Arnica has completely cured my condition but oh the joy of soothing instant relief after a massage with Arnica. The whole arm is much less painful."

Various

Linda's story:

"I went to that homeopath you recommended and he prescribed Arnica 30 and Nat Phos 6 twice daily. I was excited to find out from him that Arnica was excellent for other types of ailments as well; hypertension, digestive problems, acne, eczema, nose bleeding, tired feet, ulcers, and more. Oh, and gout! Starting Henry on Arnica straight away."

These are just a few of the many conditions Arnica can help with. There are dozens of others that users have told me helped their particular ailment. At the end of the book I have listed several resources where you can obtain more information on the wonders of Arnica therapy and more testimonials.

For first aid, homeopathic Arnica Montana is safe to use as often as is necessary and is effective for a whole range of common ailments.

There are so many ailments Arnica can help with. Keep a supply of Arnica in your home, your office, your gym bag, your car and even your suitcase!

Arnica Today

Almost every day one sees, or hears another story about Arnica in the media. Newspapers, magazines, television and radio seem to be forever digging up some new story about this or that celebrity using Arnica.

What I find exciting is that many of these stories are about findings that come from scientifically trained professionals. It is often reported that further studies are still being made in order to find even more medicinal uses of the plant.

It seems the medical community is starting to believe what we have known for decades, Arnica truly has the power to heal and relieve pain.

Like many other women I like to use Arnica for cosmetic benefits too. For example, I rinse my hair with a preparation that has Arnica flowers in it. I find it makes my hair look shiny and healthy.

Therefore I wasn't too surprised to see recent reports that some fashion designers and models in New York are taking Arnica to slim down and clear their skin before a big event. The rich and glamorous are always searching for new ways to look more beautiful. But does it work? Well I'm sure there can be benefits for the skin but I don't see how it could aid slimming.

Arnica does help reduce swelling like puffiness below the eyes, but that's hardly the same thing. It's certainly an interesting use of the herb and I look forward to seeing how the story develops.

It is reported that photographic models are using Arnica creams to combat spider veins or thread veins. What the celebrities use today, the world uses tomorrow!

Plastic surgeons all over the world advise their patients to use Arnica before and after surgery to reduce bruising and inflammation. Many cosmetic physicians use arnica themselves.

There are now facial creams containing Arnica extract, sold at Neiman Marcus for $295 for a 1.7-ounce pot!

Famous designer Linda Fargo, stylist Isabel Dupre, and Wende Zomni, the executive director of Urban Decay Cosmetics are reported users of Arnica for its excellent benefits.

Cosmetic companies are combining Arnica with additional ingredients such as olive oil, vitamin E, sunflower oil, and other herbal extractions to produce a wide range of products.

One of the world's most famous supermodels Gisele Bundchen, is said to use the Nelson Pure & Clear Acne Gel that contains Arnica extract.

At this rate of development it won't be long before most homes have some Arnica products in them. I just hope that along with the cosmetics and slimming potions everyone still keeps a bottle of homeopathic Arnica for first aid.

Arnica - Indispensible!

Herbal or Homeopathic Arnica?

It is important to understand the difference between Herbal Arnica and Arnica used in Homeopathy. Otherwise, the claims that Arnica is totally safe and the occasional warning about its use can seem contradictory.

Homeopaths believe in the power of the minimum dose, and the dilutions in Homeopathic Arnica Remedies make them completely safe.

Herbal products often use substantially higher amounts of extract from the plant and therefore in certain circumstances caution is advisable. Do not take Herbal Arnica by mouth without direct medical supervision because there can be adverse effects when taken internally. It is also not recommended to apply herbal preparations of Arnica to open wounds.

Keeping these logical cautions in mind, Arnica has been used by Herbalists for centuries and yet only an extremely small number of people have ever had adverse reactions - compare this to the thousands of people who suffer adverse drug reactions.

Making herbal products from Arnica is amazingly simple and you can even grow Arnica from seeds in your own garden. For this, you should know a couple of tips and tricks. Arnica is best grown in sandy, acidic soil. Also, the plant must receive a minimum of 6 hours of daylight. After it's harvested, you can prepare tinctures and salves from it.

Shampoos, soaps, bath soaks and skin soothers are just some of the many products that can be made. You can find instructions for making Arnica oil at anniesremedy.com, and diynatural.com has a wonderful recipe for making an Arnica salve.

Homeopathic Arnica is available in the form of tincture, ointment, cream, salve and pills. Topical gels and creams are generally rubbed on the skin at the site of pain or injury and pellets are dissolved under the tongue.

For minor, localized complaints, the topical form is recommended. For more severe general symptoms, and always in the case of associated shock, the pellet form is more effective. The little tablets can be commonly found as Arnica Montana 6 and Arnica Montana 30 but other potencies are also available.

Homeopathic medicines are delicate and should be touched as little as possible. The pellet should be put under the tongue and allowed to dissolve. It is preferable to take the dose in a 'clean mouth' and therefore at least half an hour before or after having anything to eat or drink, or cleaning your teeth.

This doesn't apply in an emergency when the dose should be taken as soon as possible. Logic also dictates that expert help is called for in all serious cases.

Herbal or homeopathic, every household should have some form of this wonder herb in their homes.

The History of Arnica

Arnica as a herbal remedy was first recognized in the British medical fraternity in the 16th century and it was added to the U.S. Pharmacopoeia in 1820.

In the last century Arnica has primarily been used by homeopaths to help heal people affected by shock, trauma or physical injuries. However it is now thought to work on the emotional level as well, reducing the effects of mental shock just as efficiently as shock to the body.

Germany's Commission E (the body tasked with evaluating the safety and efficacy of herbs for licensed medical prescribing) approved Arnica for use on the skin in treating injury and effects of accidents, any inflammation of the mouth and throat area, and insect bites.

In 2006 the British Medicines and Healthcare Products Regulatory Agency (MHRA) granted the first ever UK product registration on a traditional herbal medicinal product. The first product to be registered was Atrogel Arnica Gel.

Professor Kent Woods, Chief Executive of the MHRA said: *"This first product registration is an important landmark. We hope that Atrogel Arnica Gel will be the first of many products to receive a traditional herbal registration."*

Today Arnicas popularity is growing by leaps and bounds – according to a **New York Times** article (September 15, 2011) *'Arnica Becomes a Celebrity Favorite'.* The article quotes famous models, fashion designers and sports stars who all swear by its efficacy.

Homeopath Phyllis Speight in her excellent little book '**Arnica, The Wonder Herb'** says:

"If Arnica could be introduced into every household all over the world, countless men, women and children would be saved a vast amount of suffering."

Arnica & Homeopathic Masters

The first master of homeopathy and the one who founded and established the practice was Samuel Hahnemann, a German medical physician of the 1700s. Hahnemann experimented with Arnica and found it helped heal everything from baldness, to bruises, cramps, emotional problems, forgetfulness, gout, impotence, incontinence, sleeping problems, soreness, travel sickness, and even rheumatism.

James Tyler Kent, MD (1849 - 1916) is best remembered as a forefather of modern homeopathy in America. In his Materia Medica he found that Arnica wasn't just good for dealing with accidents and emergencies as they happen but could also be useful in chronic conditions. This is an extract: 'Arnica is useful in some chronic cases; especially in old cases of gout. It is quite a common thing for old cases of gout to rouse up into a new soreness of joints, with great sensitiveness. You will see the old grandfather sit off in a corner of the room, and if he sees little Johnnie running towards him, he will say, "Oh, do keep away, keep away." Give him a dose of Arnica and he will let Johnnie romp all over him.'

The writings of E. A. Farrington, M. D (1847 – 1885) create the impression of a master mind as well as a master homeopath. In his Clinical Materia Medica he wrote this about Arnica: 'Arnica is applicable to both the acute and chronic effects of injuries. The acute injuries for which it is useful are the following: simple bruises in which there are well-marked ecchymoses; concussions of the brain or spine, or both. We have no remedy which equals Arnica in these last-named cases. Even compression of the brain comes within the range of Arnica, whether this compression is the result of a displaced fragment of bone in cranial fracture, or the result of effusion of blood within the cranial cavity. Arnica cannot, of course, cure in the former of these cases; an operation is demanded in order to obtain permanent relief. You may use Arnica in injuries of the muscles from a strain or from a sudden wrench, as in the case of heavy lifting, and in hemorrhages of mechanical origin. Fractures of the bones may call for the use of Arnica both externally and internally to relieve the swelling and tumefaction of the limb, and also to relieve the twitching of muscles, a reflex symptom of the fracture.'

Arnica has been used and proven useful for hundreds of years. Shouldn't you be using it today?

Message from the Author

Many people who are skeptical of homeopathy say if it works at all it's only because of the placebo effect. Well, the mind is a powerful instrument and I wouldn't be surprised if many cures by alternative or mainstream medicine didn't have an element of placebo in them. And if that's the case, thank goodness for the placebo effect!

However, Arnica works particularly well with children and animals, and since they are unlikely to have rigid beliefs about illness placebo can play no part in their recovery. My faithful old Labrador was once so sore he could not walk to his food bowl, and after a dose of Arnica 30 he was running around again within minutes.

Veterinarians now use many, many treatments that are scoffed at in human medicine. Arnica, although an old, well established remedy, is not so often used as it should be in general practice. Maybe doctors treating humans could learn something from the vets!

Skeptics simply ignore personal experience, tossing it aside as if it holds no true value. And yet anecdotal evidence is routinely provided in medical journals. Why? Because such evidence does matter and every individual's personal experience does count.

Perhaps someday there will be a clear scientific explanation for how this plant works its magic. Until then, the overwhelming anecdotal evidence that has been recorded for over a hundred years or more should satisfy all but the most blinkered die-hard skeptics.

The best way for anyone to test the efficacy of Arnica is to buy some and try the remedy. Especially those who are unfortunate to suffer any of the symptoms mentioned in this book.

By discovering the amazing benefits of Arnica for yourself, you will even become a fan of Homeopathy, just from using Arnica. Even better, arrange to see a homeopath next time you have something that nobody else can seem to fix – what have you got to lose?

Arnica works…period. And remember that you can still take whatever mainstream medicine you want along with it. Homeopathy may not make sense to everyone, but it works.

I am not a homeopath, but am someone whose family has used Arnica for years and has experienced firsthand the amazing power of the little white pills. I have seen how it has helped my family and friends and read countless scores of testimonies.

Please don't deny yourself the relief and comfort that Arnica provides, waiting for scientific evidence. Arnica has changed many lives and brought healing to millions.

Let Arnica change your life for the better.

Anecdotal Evidence

Thank you so much for reading my book, I do hope you found it interesting and helpful.

It is my ambition to build up an overwhelming body of anecdotal evidence in support of the healing properties of Arnica.

Anecdotal evidence is how most knowledge has been developed throughout history. How best to do anything was figured out by seeing what worked, and then passing that information to others. People learned that certain herbs had curative value by first trying and then handing their experiences down through generations, as anecdotal evidence.

I believe the medical testimony of others truly counts as evidence and I would really like to know your experience of Arnica. Not just positive experiences, I would even like to know in what circumstances Arnica didn't work for you.

I hope you agree that all experiences, from the widest source possible, will provide valuable information on which others can base health decisions. If you do, please share yours.

If you have an anecdote about Arnica you would like to share, please help me by sending it to: anecdotes@betterlifebooks.co.za or go back to Amazon and leave your story there.

I promise to send a free copy of my next book 'About Bach Flower Remedies' to everyone who sends or leaves an anecdote.

 Best wishes in health!

Ruth Elston 2012.

References

http://www.Arnica.com/

Colin Jackson interview by Angus Watson of the London Financial Times.

Arnica Becomes a Celebrity Favorite - the NYT Style section. http://www.nytimes.com/2011/09/15/fashion/Arnica-becomes-a-celebrity-favorite-skin-deep.html

Phyllis Speight: Arnica the Wonder Herb. – Health Science Press 1977

Professor Rudolf Fritz Weiss (1895-1991) - highly regarded as the "founding father" of modern German phytotherapy.

Does Arnica really work? "can millions of patients be wrong" by Anastasia Stephens, Daily Mail.

Read more: http://www.dailymail.co.uk/health/article-160090/Does-Arnica-really-work.html#ixzz27Nba1BGD

http://www.mhra.gov.uk/NewsCentre/Pressreleases/CON2025160

Lectures On Homœopathic Materia Medica By James Tyler Kent, A.M., M.D. (1849 - 1916)

Lectures On Clinical Materia Medica By E. A. Farrington, M. D (1847 - 1885)

Blumenthal, M., P.D. Werner R. Busse, et al., Eds. (1998). The complete German Commission E Monographs. Therapeutic Guide to Herbal Medicines. Boston, MA, American Botanical Council.

Anecdotal Evidence: The Basis of All Knowledge | Gaia Health by Heidi Stevenson

Disclaimer

The information contained in this guide is not presented by a medical practitioner and is not designed to replace or take the place of any form of medicine or professional medical advice. You should consult your doctor, veterinarian or get other professional medical advice before using any of the suggested remedies in this guide.

This guide has been provided for educational and informative purposes only. All links in this report are for information purposes only and are not warranted for content, accuracy or any other implied or explicit purpose.

In self-help books, as in life, there are no guarantees of results. Readers are cautioned to rely on their own good judgment about their individual circumstances and act accordingly.

HOW TO USE TEA TREE OIL

90 Great Ways to Use Natures "Medicine Cabinet in a Bottle"

An Easy To Follow A-Z of Tea Tree Oil Uses.

How to use Tea Tree Oil includes practical advice and directions on treating a whole range of medical conditions - together with a surprisingly large number of non-medical uses; from removing bubblegum to cleaning cell phones.

- Just a few of things you will learn in this book:
- How to use Tea Tree Oil as a natural treatment for Acne
- How to destroy Head Lice
- How to cure Athletes Foot & Jock Itch
- How to use Tea Tree Oil for Bad Breath
- Awesome uses for Tea Tree Oil in the home & office
- How to cure a Cold Sore quickly
- How to use Tea Tree Oil as Insect Repellent
- How you can use Tea Tree Oil as an antiseptic to be used on Cuts and Burns
- How as an anti-viral Tea Tree Oil helps to lessen the symptoms of Colds and Flu
- How to a make a vaporizer to loosen Chest Congestion
- How to rid yourself of Dandruff and Dry Scalp!

- How to get rid of a Sinus Infection!
- How to remove Planter Warts and Skin Tags with Tea Tree Oil
- Why Tea Tree Oil is the Perfect Treatment for Fungus, Bacteria, and much, much more

This practical little guide also includes suggestions on which carrier oils to mix with Tea Tree oil; oils that when used together can improve the potency and effectiveness of both.

You will learn the correct dilutions for the different applications of the oil and how you can make your own tea tree oil products that will save you a fortune on the cost of 'over the counter' products.

If you have heard about Tea Tree Oil and have wondered what it is and how it can be used, this is *THE* book to read.

HOW TO USE TEA TREE OIL
RUTH ELSTON
ISBN 978-0-620-57247-7

Available from Amazon & all good booksellers.

Made in United States
Orlando, FL
14 June 2022

18782943R00028